How to Make Liposomal Vitamin C at Home

Complete Beginners Guide. Supercharge Your Immune System during Quarantine with Your Homemade Liposomal Vitamin C Recipes and Discover Its Uses and Benefits

Fiona Jones

Table of Contents

Introduction

What is Vitamin C?

Vitamin C, otherwise called ascorbic acid, has a few significant capacities.

These include:

- assisting with protecting cells and keeps them healthy
- keeping up healthy skin, veins, bones, and cartilage
- assisting with wound recuperating

The absence of vitamin C can prompt scurvy. Mild insufficiencies may happen in babies given unsupplemented dairy animals' milk and in individuals with poor or extremely restricted diets.

Great wellsprings of vitamin C

Nutrient C is found in a wide assortment of products of the soil.

Great sources include:

- oranges and squeezed orange
- red and green peppers
- strawberries
- blackcurrants
- broccoli
- Brussels sprout
- potatoes

What amount of vitamin C do I need?

Adults matured 19 to 64 need 40mg of vitamin C daily.

You ought to have the option to get all the vitamin C you need from your everyday diet.

Vitamin C can't be put away in the body, so you need it in your eating routine consistently.

What occurs if I take an excessive amount of vitamin C?

Taking a large amount (more than 1,000mg every day) of vitamin C can cause:

- stomach pain
- diarrhea
- fart

These side effects ought to vanish once you quit taking vitamin C supplements.

What does the Department of Health and Social Care advice?

You ought to have the option to get all the vitamin C you need by eating a differed and adjusted eating routine.

If you take vitamin C supplements, don't accept a lot as this could be destructive.

Taking under 1,000mg of vitamin C supplements a day is probably not going to bring about any harm.

Chapter 1

Why Liposomal Vitamin C?

There's little uncertainty that vitamin C is of incredible advantage to the human body. Nonetheless, how you devour vitamin C has an immense effect on the sum your body can retain and utilize (a component of all enhancements called "bioavailability").

Liposomal (or master liposomal) vitamin C is a historic choice for high-portion vitamin C.

Between 14-30% of the vitamin C expended in supplement, the structure is consumed by the body. That number can shift extraordinarily relying upon your own vitamin C needs and the kind of supplement you take. Expending five servings of raw nourishments high in vitamin C every day, for example, berries, kiwi, broccoli and citrus, will give around 200 mg of vitamin C. Including supplemental vitamin C as ascorbic acid, the proportionate type of vitamin C discovered normally in nourishments, will expand blood levels further, yet characteristic ingestion of vitamin C over intake of around 200 mg diminishes forcefully by half. This might be because our bodies utilize certain transporters of vitamin C in the small digestive tract called Sodium-Dependent Vitamin C Transporters (SVCT - 1) which will ingest proficiently just in a specific way. What's more any abundance retained vitamin C becomes discharged in pee to keep up a little tight control on plasma concentrations. This is the place liposomal vitamin C has a favorable position.

Liposomes are phospholipid containing microscopic spheres that convey vitamin C at their center. Their ingestion doesn't rely upon vitamin C transporters like SVCT-1 yet rather on direct combination of the liposome with the little intestinal cells bringing about direct intracellular arrival of the vitamin C and in the end into the blood circulation.

Not exclusively does liposomal vitamin C have a considerably higher assimilation rate than regular vitamin C supplements, it accompanies its host of medical advantages. This is because of the phospholipids it uses to encompass, or epitomize, the vitamin C — the very system that permits it to sidestep the moderate vitamin C transporters present in the gut.

What are liposomes?

Liposomes are really like cells. Similar phospholipids that makeup cells likewise make up the external shell of liposomes. The internal and external dividers of the liposome are comprised of phospholipids, the most well-known being phosphatidylcholine, to make a lipid bilayer. A twofold layer of phospholipids (phospholipid bilayer) makes a circle around a fluid (water-containing) part, for example, broke up vitamin C.

Since the liposomes' external shells mimic our phone layers, liposomes can "fuse" with specific cells upon contact, conveying the liposome's substance to the cell. This is the scientific advantage of the liposomal delivery system.

Liposomes were found during the 1960s, yet scientists have just started to expose their far-reaching applications. This novel delivery system offers a focused on technique to get supplements into the circulatory system without being devastated by the stomach related compounds and acid found in the digestive tract and stomach individually.

What is liposomal vitamin C?

On account of liposomal vitamin C (otherwise called liposomal C), these phospholipids typify vitamin C at their center.

Liposomes are thought to fuse with the cells answerable for engrossing supplements making up the gut lining called enterocytes. Since they bypass the ordinary system of engrossing vitamin C through vitamin C receptors type 1 (sodium subordinate vitamin C receptors SCVT 1), the bioavailability is a lot higher than standard vitamin C supplements.

Taking a liposomal type of nutrient C is considerably more compelling and productive than conventional strategies for nutrient C supplementation regarding ingestion.

5 Benefits of Liposomal Vitamin C

Taking standard vitamin C (ascorbic acid) offers a few advantages to the human body. These advantages might be amplified when taking liposomal C.

1. Bioavailability

The best comprehended favorable position is that liposomal vitamin C has a lot higher bioavailability than standard vitamin C.

Bioavailable essentially implies how well it ingests into your framework. As we previously referenced liposomal vitamin C supplement permits your small intestine to ingest a greater amount of the supplement than a standard enhancement.

A recent report in 11 human subjects found that vitamin C epitomized in liposomes expanded vitamin C levels in the blood by over half contrasted with an un-encapsulated (non-liposomal) supplement at a similar portion (4 grams).

Liposomal vitamin C's bioavailability is just overwhelmed by intravenous (IV) vitamin C. IV nutrient C which has 100% bioavailability by definition, however, it is significantly more obtrusive, as it requires a needle addition, a uniquely prepared office, and 1-3 hours for the slow infusion.

High portions of IV vitamin C are utilized most regularly related to malignant growth treatment and give a pro-oxidant impact which must be accomplished with exceptionally high IV dosages of vitamin C. The pro-oxidant impact of high portion IV vitamin C is different than that of low dosages of vitamin C which give hostile to oxidant activity.

2. Heart and Brain Health

Vitamin C intake (using diet or enhancements) may diminish the risk of cardiovascular disease by about 25%, as per a 2004 examination distributed in The American Journal of Clinical Nutrition.

Any type of vitamin C supplement improves endothelial capacity, just as ejection fraction.

Endothelial capacity includes the constriction and unwinding of veins, enzymatic release to oversee blood coagulating, invulnerability, and platelet adhesion. Ejection function characterizes "the level of blood that is siphoned (or ejected) out of the ventricles" when the heart contracts on each beat.

Together, these outcomes propose that vitamin C may have a significant influence on the counteraction of cardiovascular disease and the improvement of heart wellbeing.

After a stroke or cardiovascular failure, it's critical to recuperate the tissues harmed by the absence of oxygen. When the bloodstream is reestablished, the reoxygenation of beforehand oxygen-denied cells prompts harm to tissues called reperfusion, joined by "excessive generation of free radicals".

Vitamin C is a potent antioxidant that can check and kill the oxidative stress brought about by reperfusion when conveyed intravenously.

In one animal study, liposomal vitamin C forestalled brain tissue harm from reperfusion when regulated before the bloodstream was limited.

Even though blood levels accomplished by IV injected vitamin C are a lot higher than liposomal vitamin C, one examination saw that liposomal vitamin C was almost as successful as IV vitamin C at forestalling tissue damage during reperfusion. The exploration was directed in 11 subjects who had transitory hindrance of blood flow to their arms bloodstream by the tourniquet.

3. Cancer

Intravenous vitamin C can be utilized in high portions to fight cancer with traditional chemotherapy. It may not kill disease all alone, yet it can improve personal satisfaction, expanding vitality and state of mind for some cancer patients.

Dependent upon the situation, IV vitamin C can even actuate relapse of malignant growth. A 2014 survey relates a few reports of remission when utilizing IV nutrient C with chemotherapy.

In any case, one ought not to depend on IV vitamin C to incite abatement or treat cancer all alone, as these cases are detached, best case scenario.

Liposomal vitamin C has not been explicitly tried in human subjects with cancer. Numerous cancer patients accepting adjunctive IV vitamin C, however, likewise use liposomal vitamin C in high portions between IV medicines. In the wake of getting a high portion of IV vitamin C, it isn't extraordinary for blood levels to dip under ordinary in the days after the mixture. Consequently, it's strongly prescribed to build oral intake levels of vitamin C between IV vitamin C imbuements particularly to prevent low bounce back through plasma levels of vitamin C.

4. Collagen Production

Collagen is the most bottomless protein in the Animal Kingdom, however, our body's normal collagen creation eases back around the age of 25. Vitamin C is a cofactor in the compounds that produce collagen, which means it is important to the capacity and health of your bones, veins, and joints where collagen abounds.

5. Oxidative Stress

By and large, some degree of oxidative stress happens inside each living thing. As a 2006 review put it:

"There is expanding proof interfacing oxidative worry with an assortment of neurotic conditions including malignant growth, cardiovascular sicknesses, chronic inflammatory disease, post-ischaemic organ injury, diabetes mellitus, xenobiotic/drug toxicity, and rheumatoid arthritis."

Vitamin C is powerful cell reinforcement and is found in liberal amounts inside the human body.

Although the utilization of standard cancer prevention agent supplements, similar to vitamin C, should fill in as compelling insurance against oxidative stress, there is little proof that it has a noteworthy effect in the resulting cellular damage.

Is liposomal vitamin C really powerful?

There has been a great deal of investigation of liposomal vitamin C.

One of the most now and again posed inquiries about liposomal supplements is: Is liposomal vitamin C a "lie"?

Genuine liposomal or professional liposomal supplements are non-dangerous and can significantly expand your body's capacity to retain the supplements inside. Given broad hardware and innovation expected to make them, liposomal supplements will, in general, be more costly than customary nutrient C. Be that as it may, they do convey predominant assimilation.

In any case, how would we know which items are "genuine" powerful liposomal vitamin C?

The expression "liposomal" isn't all around characterized, however, instead of the expression "liposome".

A liposome is a circular structure made out of a shell-shaped by phospholipids and encompassed by water. At the focal point of a "liposome" is normally a fundamental fixing, similar to nutrient C or glutathione, likewise suspended in water.

"Liposomal" doesn't signify "liposome" — these terms are not indeed the very same. The term liposomal is now and then approximately used to signify "containing fat".

Given this, a few items marked as "liposomal" vitamin C don't use "liposome" delivery by any stretch of the imagination. Rather, they contain a lipid (fat) and some vitamin C. The lipid structure that a few enhancements use isn't even a phospholipid, they can just be as unsaturated fat.

These structures are marked "liposomal" vitamin C yet may never bring about framed liposomes, when presented to water because the vitamin C is essentially covalently bound to unsaturated fat, no a phospholipid, which is the atom customarily expected to shape a lipid bi-layer when presented to water.

An ideal case of this is an ester of vitamin C (generally named as lipid "solvent" nutrient C) is promoted as a "liposomal" supplement that infers higher retention.

Ascorbyl palmitate is one such model. It ties palmitate (an ester) to vitamin C (ascorbic acid). This cancer prevention agent is regularly used to expand the timeframe of the realistic usability of specific nourishments, meds, and beauty care products.

Anyway ester types of vitamin C, as ascorbyl palmitate, are completely processed after oral ingestion by catalysts in the small digestive system which sever the bond promptly releasing increase outright vitamin C (ascorbic corrosive particle) and the ester, right now, before any assimilation can happen. Since plain vitamin C is framed from the ester, no improved assimilation happens when contrasted with a standard vitamin C supplement.

The esters utilized may even have a negative effect, contingent upon the ingredient itself.

Not at all like ascorbic acid, ascorbyl palmitate may be lethal to skin cells harmed by UV exposure. Its bioavailability is indistinguishable from ascorbic acid alone.

Ascorbyl oleate is fundamentally the same as the previous compound, restricting oleate to ascorbic corrosive. Almost no is thought about cetyl ascorbate other than that it is esterified vitamin C.

The reality is this: These "lipid-soluble" structures are not actually "liposomal" vitamin C and may not offer the advantages of ingestion similarly as obvious liposomal conveyance. Sadly, this outcome in unassuming clients paying as much as possible for an item that is the same as a standard vitamin C container or powder.

Along these lines, to address the inquiry: Liposomal vitamin C isn't a "hoax", however not all items named liposomal vitamin C genuinely offer similar advantages.

The most effective method to Choose the Best Liposomal Vitamin C Supplement

A few brands offer liposomal vitamin C supplements. Which vitamin liposomal nutrient C supplement is the best?

There are two fundamental sorts of liposomal supplements. The first is a formed liposome, while the other is a pro liposome.

The easiest method to tell if an item is a framed liposome is if the fixings incorporate water. If water is in the fixings, you are likely managing shaped liposomes.

A genius liposome can turn into a liposome when presented to water, compelling the phospholipids to promptly assemble by common hydrophobic powers into a bi-layer as portrayed previously.

A pro liposome can come as a powder or a fluid.

As a powder, vitamin C is encompassed (conjugated) by a layer of phospholipids and different fats in a unique specialized procedure that can extraordinarily fluctuate inadequacy. How well this exclusive procedure of restricting the lipids to the vitamin C happens is critical, supposing that the lipids and the vitamin C are just combined (not bound), the arrangement of liposomes with vitamin C inside will be sporadic, best case scenario as the vitamin C can simply scatter away independently from the lipids.

Liquid pro liposomes use lipids (fats) and vitamin C. Given extraordinary assembling strategies, the lipids structure liposomes around the fundamental fixing when they are presented to water and right temperature conditions, as are discovered nature of the small digestive system.

The recently shaped liposomes would then be able to be consumed by the intestinal dividers, conveyed to and prepared by the liver, and released into the systemic circulation.

These formed liposomes or pro liposomes use phospholipids, phosphatidylcholine, lecithin, and oleic acid (or a mix of all) as the greasy operator to frame liposomes.

Tragically, numerous vitamin C supplements named "liposomal" are, actually, incapable to hold the lipid fixing and vitamin C together when presented to water in the small digestive system.

Ensure the vitamin C is very much sourced. A decent liposomal vitamin C supplement ought to be non-GMO and ideally use phospholipids got from sunflower lecithin.

A few clients even demand to realize that the cause of vitamin C is non-Chinese.

Quali-C brand vitamin C is one such source, made in Scotland from non-GMO European cause corn.

At last, just try liposomal nutrient C that has a fulfillment ensure with a full refund on the occasion you aren't content with the item.

To outline: Avoid the tricks and buy an excellent liposomal supplement by following these means:

1. Pick a framed liposomal or a very much made pro liposomal supplement that contains vitamin C and a fatty substance (phospholipids or phosphatidylcholine), yet does exclude ascorbyl palmitate, ascorbyl oleate, or cetyl ascorbate as they offer no preferred position over regular vitamin C.
2. Search for a dose of around 1,000 mg/day.

3. Guarantee the enhancement is non-GMO and soy-, gluten-, and artificial preservative-free.
4. Avoid items sourced in China.
5. Search for organizations that have positive surveys and offer a robust refund policy.

Dosages of Liposomal Vitamin C

The National Institute of Health prompts people to never take more than 2,000 milligrams of vitamin C dietary enhancement every day.

For explicit medical problems, a higher portion might be justified. The Linus Pauling Center prescribes a portion of 2,000 milligrams for every day, which is protected and can represent more unfortunate retention limits in certain people. Individuals that may profit most from this high portion incorporate the old and smokers, who have an expanded requirement for vitamin C.

By and large, 1000-2000 mg/day ought to manage the cost of you the general health benefits of vitamin C:

- Invulnerability
- Cerebrum wellbeing
- Collagen creation
- Cardiovascular production
- Energy creation
- Expanded cancer prevention agent nearness

4,000 milligrams of liposomal vitamin C have been utilized to ensure against the oxidative harm that can happen post-cardiovascular failure or stroke because of reperfusion.

While these outcomes are exceptionally encouraging, I recommend staying at or underneath the 2,000-milligram edge except if a medicinal services professional encourages you to take a higher sum, even though the reactions of taking bigger portions are not risky.

Liposomal Vitamin C Side Effects

Albeit a high portion of vitamin C may not, in fact, be "lethal", it might cause symptoms like sickness or diarrhea.

Medication Interactions

Vitamin C connects with specific medications or supplements.

ADD and ADHD medications use amphetamines. Vitamin C may debilitate the impact of amphetamine-based medications by restricting their impact, although this outcome has not been replicated in human subjects.

In Summary

- Liposomal vitamin C is a progressive way to deal with bringing vitamin C into your framework.
- Liposomes utilize a phospholipid bilayer conformed to water and, right now, C. The external packaging shields the supplement inside from harm that may somehow or another happen during typical assimilation.
- The assimilation of liposomal vitamin C is altogether higher than that of a standard vitamin C supplement.
- Advantages of liposomal vitamin C incorporate expanded bioavailability, cardiovascular help, skin wellbeing, cancer protection, expanded collagen creation, and decreased oxidative worry all through the body.
- While numerous enhancements are named as "liposomal," a portion of these utilization esters of nutrient C (ascorbyl palmitate, ascorbyl oleate, or potentially cetyl ascorbate) that don't build the bioavailability of nutrient C and are false "liposomal" or "ace liposomal" items.
- Standard dosages of vitamin C are between 200-1,000 mg/day. We prescribe 1000-2000 mg for every day.

Chapter 2

How much vitamin C do people need?

Vitamin C is a water-solvent supplement with numerous essential functions in your body.

It fortifies your immune system, helps collagen creation and wound mending, and goes about as a cancer prevention agent to shield your cells from free radical damage.

Vitamin C is otherwise called L-ascorbic acid, or just ascorbic acid.

In contrast to different animals, people can't synthesize vitamin C all alone. Subsequently, you should get enough of it from nourishments or enhancements to keep up good health.

This clarifies the suggested dose of vitamin C for ideal wellbeing.

What's the suggested intake?

The Institute of Medicine (IOM) has built up a lot of reference value for explicit supplement consumption levels, including vitamin C.

One lot of rules are known as the Recommended Dietary Allowance (RDA) and considers normal day by day nutrient intake from the two nourishments and enhancements.

RDA proposals for explicit specific gender and age groups should meet the supplement needs of 97–98% of sound people

Notwithstanding the RDA suggestions for vitamin C, the Food and Drug Administration (FDA) has given a prescribed Daily Value (DV).

The DV was created for nourishment and supplement names. It causes you to decide the level of supplements in a solitary serving of nourishment, contrasted and the everyday prerequisites. On food labels, this is shown as %DV.

As of now, the suggested DV for vitamin C for adults and kids matured 4 or more is 60 mg regardless of gender.

The RDA for Vitamin C ranges from 15–75 mg for kids, 75 mg for adult women, 90 mg for adult men, and 85–120 mg for women who are pregnant or breastfeeding.

May profit a few conditions

Vitamin C is basic for in general wellbeing and health, and the supplement may especially profit certain conditions.

The vitamin is particularly useful for insusceptible wellbeing, as it underpins your invulnerable framework's cell work.

For example, vitamin C enhancements may help forestall contamination, while an insufficiency of the vitamin seems to make you increasingly powerless to disease.

For instance, some examination recommends that albeit standard vitamin C intake likely won't keep you from contracting a bug, it might decrease the length or seriousness of cold symptoms.

A review of 31 examinations found that devouring 1–2 grams of vitamin C daily reduced the cold length by 18% in children and 8% in adults.

Also, it's realized that nutrient C builds iron absorption. Subsequently, people with iron lack may profit by expanding their vitamin C intake.

Consistently getting 1–2 grams of vitamin C every day may diminish the span of normal cold side effects and lift your invulnerable framework. It may likewise help forestall iron insufficiency anemia.

Best food sources

Ordinarily, the best wellsprings of vitamin C are fruits and vegetables.

Note that vitamin C in nourishment is effectively obliterated by heat, however since numerous great wellsprings of the supplement are products of the soil, essentially eating a portion of those nourishments crude is a simple method to arrive at the suggested intake.

For instance, a 1/2-cup (75-gram) serving of raw red pepper gives 158% of the RDA set by the IOM.

The table beneath shows the vitamin c content and commitment to the suggested Daily Value (DV) for probably the best nourishment wellsprings of the supplement.

This table depends on the present 60-mg suggestion, however since any nourishment giving 20% or a greater amount of the DV for vitamin C is viewed as a high source, a significant number of these nourishments will even now be incredible sources after the DV proposal.

Good food sources of vitamin c include:

Food	Amount per serving	%DV
Red pepper, 1/2 cup (75 grams)	95 mg	158%
Orange juice, 3/4 cup (177 ml)	93 mg	155%
Kiwifruit, 1/2 cup (90 grams)	64 mg	107%
Green pepper, 1/2 cup (75 grams)	60 mg	100%
Broccoli, cooked, 1/2 cup (78 grams)	51 mg	85%
Strawberries, fresh, 1/2 cup (72 grams)	49 mg	82%
Brussels sprouts, cooked, 1/2 cup (81 grams)	48 mg	80%

The best nourishment wellsprings of vitamin C are fruits and vegetables. The supplement is effectively demolished by heat, so devouring these nourishments crude may boost your nutrient intake.

Best vitamin C supplements

When searching for a nutrient C supplement, you may see the supplement in a couple of various structures:

- ascorbic acid
- mineral ascorbates, for example, sodium ascorbate and calcium ascorbate
- ascorbic acid with bioflavonoids

Picking an enhancement with ascorbic acid is normally a good decision, as it has a significant level of bioavailability, which means your body retains it effectively.

Furthermore, given that most multivitamins contain ascorbic acid, picking a multivitamin won't just lift your vitamin C intake yet additionally your admission of different supplements.

To guarantee you're accepting sufficient measures of vitamin C from the enhancement you pick, search for an enhancement that gives between 45–120 mg of this vitamin relying upon your age and sex.

Vitamin C supplements arrive in an assortment of structures. Pick an enhancement with ascorbic acid to make it simpler for your body to ingest the supplement.

Would you be able to take excessively?

Although vitamin C has a general low poisonous quality risk in sound people, expending a lot of it can cause some antagonistic gastrointestinal side effects, including spasms, queasiness, and the runs.

Also, since a high vitamin C intake builds the body's assimilation of non-heme iron, expending an excessive amount of vitamin C could mess up individuals with hemochromatosis, a condition where the body holds an excess of iron.

To avoid gastrointestinal symptoms, keep your vitamin C intake inside the ULs set up by the IOM. People with hemochromatosis ought to be especially wary when taking vitamin C supplements.

Vitamin C is a water-soluble vitamin and basic cancer prevention agent that assumes numerous jobs in your body. It underpins wound recuperating, collagen arrangement, and immunity.

The RDA for vitamin C is 45–120 mg relying upon your age and sex.

Vitamin C enhancements should meet the RDA and remain well underneath the setup UL — 400 for small kids, 1,200 mg for kids aged 9–13, 1,800 mg for adolescents, and 2,000 mg for adults.

Devouring a variety of vitamin C-rich fruits and vegetables can likewise go far in supporting ideal wellbeing and health.

Effects of vitamin C deficiencies

Vitamin C is a basic supplement that must be expended consistently to forestall inadequacy.

While inadequacy is moderately uncommon in developed countries because of the accessibility of crisp production and the expansion of vitamin C to specific nourishments and enhancements, it despite everything influences generally 7% of adults in the US.

The most widely recognized risk factors for vitamin C deficiency are alcohol addiction, anorexia, serious dysfunctional behavior, smoking, and dialysis.

While manifestations of serious nutrient C insufficiency can take a very long time to create, there are some unpretentious signs to look out for.

Here are the 15 most basic signs and symptoms of vitamin C deficiency.

1. Unpleasant, Bumpy Skin

Vitamin C assumes a key job in collagen creation, a protein that is bounteous in connective tissues like skin, hair, joints, bones, and veins.

At the point when vitamin C levels are low, a skin condition known as keratosis pilaris can create.

Right now, "chicken skin" frames on the rear of the upper arms, thighs or bum because of the development of keratin protein inside the pores.

Keratosis pilaris brought about by vitamin C deficiency ordinarily shows up following three to five months of insufficient intake and resolves with supplementation.

In any case, there are numerous other potential reasons for keratosis pilaris, so its essence alone isn't sufficient to analyze an inadequacy.

Vitamin C insufficiency can cause the arrangement of small acne-like bumps on the arms, thighs or backside. Notwithstanding, these bumps alone are insufficient to analyze and inadequacy.

2. Corkscrew-Shaped Body Hair

Vitamin C deficiency can likewise make hair develop in bowed or coiled shapes because of imperfections that create in the protein structure of hair as it develops.

Corkscrew-shaped hair is one of the trademark indications of vitamin C lack yet may not be self-evident, as these damped hairs are bound to dampen off or drop out.

Hair abnormalities from the norm regularly resolve inside one month of treatment with sufficient measures of vitamin C.

Strangely bowed, curled or corkscrew-formed body hairs are a hallmark indication of vitamin C inadequacy, yet they might be hard to recognize, as these hairs are bound to drop out.

3. Bright Red Hair Follicles

Hair follicles on the outside of the skin contain numerous small veins that supply blood and supplements to the zone.

At the point when the body is inadequate in vitamin C, these little veins become delicate and break effectively, causing little, splendid red spots to show up around the hair follicles.

This is known as perifollicular hemorrhage and a very much recorded indication of extreme vitamin C deficiency.

Taking vitamin C supplements normally settle this side effect inside about fourteen days.

Hair follicles contain tiny blood veins that can crack because of a vitamin C insufficiency, making splendid red spots show up around the follicles.

4. Spoon-Shaped Fingernails with Red Spots or Lines

Spoon-shaped nails are described by their sunken shape and regularly dainty and weak. They are all the more normally connected with iron inadequacy weakness however have additionally been connected to vitamin C deficiency.

Red spots or vertical lines in the nail bed, known as fragment discharge, may likewise show up during vitamin c deficiency because of debilitated veins that burst no problem at all.

While the visual appearance of fingernails and toenails may help decide the probability of nutrient C insufficiency, note that it's not viewed as demonstrative.

Vitamin C deficiency is related to spoon-molded fingernails and red lines or spots underneath the nail bed.

5. Dry, Damaged Skin

Healthy skin contains a lot of vitamin C, particularly in the epidermis, or external layer of skin.

Vitamin C keeps skin health by shielding it from oxidative harm brought about by the sun and introduction to contaminations like tobacco smoke or the ozone.

It additionally advances collagen creation, which keeps skin looking full and young.

High intake of vitamin C is related to better skin quality, while lower intake is related to a 10% expanded risk of creating dry, wrinkled skin.

While dry, harmed skin can be connected to vitamin C deficiency, it can likewise be brought about by numerous different elements, so this side effect alone isn't sufficient to analyze an inadequacy.

Low intake of vitamin C is related to dry, sun-harmed skin, yet these side effects can likewise be brought about by different components.

6. Simple Bruising

Wounding happens when veins under the skin crack, making blood spill into the encompassing regions.

Simple wounding is a typical indication of vitamin C inadequacy since poor collagen creation causes weak blood vessels.

Deficiency related wounds may cover huge zones of the body or show up as little, purple spots under the skin.

Easy bruising is regularly one of the clear side effects of a lack and should warrant further examination concerning vitamin C levels.

Vitamin C inadequacy debilitates veins, causing simple wounding. It's regularly one of the primary clear indications of vitamin C lack.

7. Gradually Healing Wounds

Since vitamin C lack eases back the pace of collagen development, it makes wounds recuperate all the more gradually.

Research has demonstrated that individuals with interminable, non-recuperating leg ulcers are altogether bound to be insufficient in vitamin C than those without incessant leg ulcers.

In extreme instances of vitamin C insufficiency, old injuries may even revive, expanding the risk of infection.

Slow twisted healing is one of the further developed indications of lack and commonly not seen until somebody has been inadequate for a long time.

Vitamin C deficiency meddles with tissue development, making wounds mend all the more gradually. This is viewed as a propelled indication of inadequacy, so different signs and side effects would almost certainly show up first.

8. Painful, Swollen Joints

Since joints contain a great deal of collagen-rich connective tissue, they can likewise be influenced by vitamin C deficiency.

There have been many revealed instances of joint pain related to vitamin C insufficiency, frequently extreme enough to cause limping or difficulty walking.

Bleeding inside the joints can likewise happen in individuals who are lacking in vitamin C, causing growing and extra pain.

However, both of these symptoms can be treated with vitamin C supplements and ordinarily resolve inside multi-week.

Vitamin C inadequacy regularly causes serious joint agony. In extreme cases, draining can happen inside the joints, causing painful swallowing.

9. Weak Bones

Vitamin C inadequacy can likewise influence bone wellbeing. Indeed, low intake has been connected to the expanded risk of crack and osteoporosis.

Research has discovered that vitamin C assumes a basic job in bone formation, so an insufficiency can expand the pace of bone misfortune.

Youngsters' skeletons might be particularly influenced by nutrient C insufficiency, as they are as yet developing and creating.

Vitamin C is significant for bone formation, and inadequacy can increase the risk of creating brittle and weak bones.

10. Bleeding Gums and Tooth Loss

Red, swollen, bleeding gums are another basic indication of vitamin C deficiency.

Without satisfactory vitamin C, gum tissue gets debilitated and excited and veins drain all the more effectively.

In advance stages of vitamin C deficiency, gums may even seem purple and spoiled.

In the long run, teeth can drop out because of undesirable gums and frail dentin, the calcified internal layer of teeth.

Red, bleeding gums are a typical indication of vitamin C insufficiency, and serious lack can even prompt tooth loss.

11. Poor Immunity

Studies show that vitamin C amasses inside different kinds of insusceptible cells to assist them with combatting contamination and demolish ailment causing pathogens.

Vitamin C lack is related to poor invulnerability and a higher risk of infection, including genuine ailments like pneumonia.

Numerous individuals with scurvy, an ailment brought about by vitamin C deficiency, in the end, bite the dust of infection because of their poorly function immune system.

Vitamin C is a significant vitamin for the insusceptible framework. Low vitamin C levels are connected to an increased risk of infection, while serious inadequacy can cause demise from the irresistible disease.

12. Persistent Iron Deficiency Anemia

Vitamin C and iron insufficiency weakness frequently happen together.

Signs of iron insufficiency frailty incorporate whiteness, exhaustion, inconvenience breathing during exercise, dry skin and hair, cerebral pain and spoon-formed fingernails.

Low degrees of vitamin C may add to press inadequacy paleness by diminishing the ingestion of iron from plant-based nourishments and contrarily influencing iron digestion.

Vitamin C inadequacy additionally expands the risk of over the top dying, which can add to anemia.

If iron insufficiency anemia continues for quite a while with no conspicuous causes, it might be wise to check your vitamin C levels.

Vitamin C deficiency may expand the danger of iron inadequacy weakness by lessening iron assimilation and improving the probability of bleeding.

13. Fatigue and Poor Mood

Two of the most punctual indications of vitamin C deficiency are weakness and poor disposition.

These side effects can even show up before an all-out inadequacy creates.

While fatigue and touchiness might be a portion of the main indications to show up, they regularly resolve after only a couple of long periods of sufficient intake or inside 24 hours of high-portion supplementation.

Indications of fatigue and poor mind-set can show up even with low-to-ordinary degrees of vitamin C, yet they rapidly pivot with satisfactory vitamin C intake.

14. Unexplained Weight Gain

Vitamin C may help ensure against obesity by directing the arrival of fat from fat cells, diminishing pressure hormones and diminishing inflammation.

Research has discovered a reliable connection between low intake of vitamin C and abundance muscle versus fat, yet it's not satisfactory whether it is circumstances and logical results relationship.

Strikingly, low blood levels of vitamin C have been connected to higher measures of tummy fat, even in ordinary weight people.

While abundance muscle versus fat alone isn't sufficient to demonstrate a vitamin C lack, it might merit looking at after different variables have been precluded.

Low vitamin C intake has been connected to expanded muscle versus fat in people, yet different variables might be included, for example, diet quality.

15. Chronic Inflammation and Oxidative Stress

Vitamin C is one of the body's most significant water-solvent cancer prevention agents.

It forestalls cell harm by killing free radicals that can cause oxidative pressure and irritation in the body.

Oxidative pressure and inflammation have been connected to numerous incessant sicknesses, including coronary illness and diabetes, so lessening levels are likely helpful.

Low intake of vitamin C has been connected to more significant levels of aggravation and oxidative worry, just as an expanded risk of coronary illness.

One investigation found that grown-ups with the most minimal blood levels of vitamin C were about 40% bound to create cardiovascular breakdown inside 15 years than those with the most noteworthy blood levels, even though they were not inadequate in vitamin C.

Normal utilization of cell reinforcements like vitamin C is related to medical advantages, while low intake may expand aggravation and oxidative pressure.

The Best Food Sources of Vitamin C

The recommended daily intake (RDI) for vitamin C is 90 mg for men and 75 mg for women.

Smokers are encouraged to expend an extra 35 mg for every day, as tobacco diminishes the retention of vitamin C and expands the body's utilization of the supplement.

Next to no vitamin C is expected to forestall scurvy. Only 10 mg for every day is sufficient, which is generally the sum found in one tablespoon of new ringer pepper or the juice of a large portion of a lemon.

The absolute best nourishment wellsprings of vitamin C (per cup) incorporate:

Acerola cherry: 2,740% of the RDI

Guava: 628% of the RDI

Blackcurrants: 338% of the RDI

Sweet red pepper: 317% of the RDI

Kiwifruit: 273% of the RDI

Lychee: 226% of the RDI

Lemon: 187% of the RDI

Orange: 160% of the RDI

Strawberry: 149% of the RDI

Papaya: 144% of the RDI

Broccoli: 135% of the RDI

Parsley: 133% of the RDI

Vitamin C quickly separates when presented to warm, so raw products of the soil are preferable sources overcooked ones.

Since the body doesn't store a lot of vitamin C, it is prescribed to eat new foods grown from the ground each day.

Enhancing with vitamin C has not been seen as dangerous, yet taking more than 2,000 mg for every day may cause stomach issues, looseness of the bowels and queasiness, just as increment the risk of creating oxalate kidney stones in men.

Furthermore, dosages more than 250 mg for each day may meddle with tests intended to recognize blood in the stool or stomach and ought to be stopped two weeks before testing.

Fresh fruits and vegetables are brilliant wellsprings of nutrient C and ought to forestall insufficiency when expended every day. Enhancing with vitamin C isn't poisonous however may cause terrible symptoms at high portions.

Vitamin C deficiency is generally uncommon in evolved nations yet at the same time influences more than 1 out of 20 individuals.

Since people can't make vitamin C or store it in huge sums, it must be devoured normally to forestall inadequacy, preferably through crisp products of the soil.

There are numerous signs and symptoms of deficiency, a large portion of which are identified with disabilities in collagen creation or not expending enough cancer prevention agents.

The absolute soonest indications of inadequacy incorporate weakness, red gums, simple wounding and dying, joint pain and rough, bumpy skin.

As the lack of advances, bones may get weak, nail and hair disfigurements can create, wounds may take more time to recuperate and the resistant framework endures.

Aggravation, iron-inadequacy frailty and unexplained weight increase might be different signs to look for.

Fortunately, lack of side effects are normally settled once vitamin C levels are reestablished.

Chapter 3

Why liposomal supplements

Advantages of Liposomal Supplements

A healthy diet with crisp, healthy fixings makes ready for ideal wellbeing. But sometimes, for a variety of reasons, you may likewise require extra help as wellbeing supplements to get basic supplements, to address nutritional deficiencies and to improve your wellbeing. However, do these supplements truly work?

You can ingest just a specific measure of the supplements and micronutrients you get from your nourishment and supplements.

For example, resveratrol and curcumin supplements offer unbelievable medical advantages, however, they are constrained by their poor assimilation and low bioavailability. Glutathione is one of the most significant cancer prevention agents your body makes all alone, yet its creation decays with age. In this way, taking it in supplement structure is by all accounts the most consistent approach to keep up sound levels to enable your body to keep up its enemy of oxidant status. However, ordinary oral supplements are insufficient in improving glutathione levels in the blood, as a large portion of it is degraded during digestion.

Nutrients, minerals and cancer prevention agents must arrive at target cells and tissues to offer wanted medical advantages. That is the reason it is imperative to pick your enhancement in a structure that improves the retention of supplements, making them increasingly accessible to your cells. This carries us to liposomal supplements that guarantee higher ingestion and bioavailability than your typical oral supplements.

All in all, what are these liposomal supplements? Let us initially talk about what liposomes are and why these structures fill in as great transporters to convey nutrients, supplements and different operators straightforwardly to the cells and tissues in your body.

What are liposomes?

The word 'liposome' originates from two Greek words: 'Lipos', which means fat and 'Soma', which means body.

Liposomes are little estimated vesicles made of phospholipids, a class of fats that are the fundamental auxiliary part of your cell layers. A liposome has an extremely fascinating structure with an empty center encased by a phospholipid bilayer. It's this twofold layer structure that makes liposomes an exceptionally compelling vehicle to convey medications and supplements – conveying them straightforwardly into the circulation system and to your cells.

A phospholipid molecule comprises a head and a tail which are consolidated by a glycerol molecule. The head is made of phosphate gathering though the tail has two long chains of unsaturated fats. The tail, comprising of unsaturated fat chains, is hydrophobic, which means it is repulsed by water. Then again the head, made of the phosphate group is hydrophilic, which means it adores water.

The magic happens when phospholipids are scattered in water or an aqueous solution. These particles naturally mastermind themselves in one of a kind way. The water-hating lipid tail moves from the water and the water-loving phosphate head moves towards the water surface. This direction brings about the arrangement of fixed, circular structures that have an empty center encompassed by a double layer-membrane. These vesicles or air pockets are called liposomes.

Traditional forms of supplements versus liposomal supplements

Taking vitamins and mineral enhanced enhancements doesn't promise you are getting all the essential supplements you need. To get why allows first to go over a significant factor called bioavailability.

Understanding bioavailability

For a supplement to have the ideal result, it must be appropriately processed and shipped into the circulatory framework.

Bioavailability is how much supplements from nourishment and enhancements become accessible in your tissues and circulation system for prepared assimilation after they are processed. Few out of every odd nutrient, mineral or medication has the equivalent bio-accessibility. Some are rapidly and effectively assimilated, others may require extra assistance though some are not completely retained.

Bioavailability relies upon numerous components, for example,

Overall wellbeing and age:

Individuals more than 60 experience difficulty retaining most supplements, particularly nutrient B12 and magnesium.

Strength of the digestive tract:

Conditions, for example, Crohn's, celiac disease and irritable bowel syndrome (IBS) influence the retention of supplements (got through nourishment or enhancements) by the body.

Utilization of specific medications:

Medications that are utilized to treat acidity and heartburn (for instance, proton siphon inhibitors) can confine the assimilation of vitamin B12 just as minerals, for example, magnesium and iron. Metformin, a regularly utilized enemy of diabetic medication, likewise meddles with the assimilation of vitamin B12, causing B12 deficiency. Additionally, anti-infection agents wreck great microscopic organisms in the gut alongside terrible. Since you need solid microbes for appropriate processing and assimilation of supplements, delayed utilization of anti-infection agents likewise impacts bioavailability.

Collaboration with different nutrients:

Some vitamins and minerals are better ingested when they are expended alongside different supplements. This is the reason there is such a solid accentuation on eating an even, brilliant eating routine that contains all the vitamins, minerals and phytochemicals. You need vitamin C to help retain iron and magnesium to appropriately utilize nutrient D. Then again, zinc and iron ought to be taken independently as zinc is known to repress the ingestion of iron.

Different variables that influence bioavailability to incorporate the utilization of alcohol and caffeine, liver wellbeing and whether the supplement is water dissolvable or fat solvent. It additionally relies upon how your enhancement or medication is defined, regardless of whether the time has time-released, sublingual, fluid, pill, powder or liposomal. Liposomal supplements have an edge over conventional types of enhancements regarding how effectively they are assimilated and utilized by your cells.

Why traditional oral supplements have poor bioavailability?

When you take regular supplements through the mouth, a significant measure of active ingredients is separated during the procedure of digestion. The acidic environment in the stomach, stomach related compounds, and intestinal microorganisms disintegrate the supplements. Thus, just a little portion of the total nutrients you have ingested opens up for your cells to assimilate and utilize.

Likewise, a few supplements, when taken in enormous dosages or for a prolonged duration, may create stomach problems, for example, swelling, pain in the abdomen and diarrhea. This can be trying as developing proof propose that specific vitamins, for example, vitamin C, ought to be taken in higher sums (than suggested everyday dosage) if, for instance, you are hoping to use its advantages for heart health.

Advantages of utilizing liposomal supplements

Protect nutrients from disintegration and oxidation:

Liposomes form a barrier around the cargo of supplements it conveys. This boundary shields the embodied substances from being separated by the harsh chemical and organic conditions of the gastrointestinal tract. Liposomes additionally protect the supplements from the oxidative harm brought about by free radicals. Above all, this defensive shield stays flawless until the payload of supplements is conveyed to the cells.

Simple penetration into the cells:

Liposomes are made of a similar sort of fats that your cell layers are made out of – making these nanospheres good with biological membranes. This permits them to effortlessly enter the membrane barrier, without utilizing a lot of energy. A few vitamins, for example, vitamin C, are water solvent and not exceptionally powerful in infiltrating the phone layers which are fundamentally made of lipids or fats. Then again, supplements like CoQ10 are fat solvent. The beneficial thing about liposomes is that they contain both water-loving and water-repelling compartments and are in this way very valuable in shipping both fat-solvent and water-soluble nutrients.

No side-effects:

Standard enhancements are related to gastrointestinal (GI) distress, particularly when taken in high portions. Liposomal details by-pass the GI route and therefore represent no such risks.

Liposomes are not constrained to delivering nutrients and cell reinforcements, for example, vitamin C, glutathione, magnesium, curcumin and glutathione to expand their ingestion and bioavailability. Clinical trials show that liposomal delivery systems can be effectively used to deliver anti-cancer drugs, anti-infection agents, against parasitic meds, anesthetics, and anti-inflammatory drugs.

Taking liposomal enhancements can have an enormous effect on your wellbeing, as they help:

- Improve the bioavailability of nutrients
- Protect nutrients from the components of the gastrointestinal tract
- Improve the take-up and ingestion of supplements by the cells
- Convey both water-dissolvable and fat-solvent supplements effortlessly
- Limit symptoms related to normal oral enhancements

Chapter 4

Why Liposomal Supplements Are the Next Wave of Good Nutrition

We live in a period of unprecedented nourishment plenitude—simply stroll into any grocery store and you'll locate an authentic Garden of Eden, with new organic products, greens, and vegetables from around the world, just as crisply prepared entire grain bread, wild-got fish, and a panoply of yogurts created from dairy or nut milk. We likewise abound in the least expensive nourishment accessible ever during the 1930s, Americans spent a fourth of our discretionary income on nourishment while today we spend under a tenth. What's more, our decision of solid nourishments has extended—there has been a 27% expansion in the utilization of fresh fruits of the soil 21% expansion in utilization new vegetables from 1970 to 2010. We're eating more broccoli, cauliflower, tomatoes, onions, apples, bananas, and grapes.

However notwithstanding this abundance, we are frequently supplement insufficient—more than 40 percent of grown-ups have a dietary intake of vitamin A, C, D and E, calcium and magnesium below the normal necessity for their age and sexual orientation. Furthermore, these insights don't consider the significant cancer prevention agents that keep us solid, for example, glutathione, coenzyme Q10, and resveratrol.

Are standard, oral multivitamin supplements the appropriate response? Almost two out of three adults in America think since they take vitamin, mineral or natural enhancements. However, normal oral enhancement may not convey its full therapeutic potential. Enzymes in the stomach and gastrointestinal tract can debase oral enhancements. All alone, powerful cancer prevention agents will most likely be unable to productively cross cell layers. For example, various flavonoids that show intense cancer prevention agent movement in vitro in the research facility, accomplish low focus in the blood after oral consumption. One of the most steroid antioxidants, resveratrol, related with longer life expectancy, lower risk of coronary illness, and lower levels of aggravation, is ineffectively caught up in oral enhancement form. CoQ10 supplementation can be trying: as a lipid-loving (lipophilic) molecule, CoQ10 is best processed with fats and endures poor ingestion in water.

As per William Judy, author of SIBR Research, under 1 percent of basic CoQ10 powder is assimilated. Correspondingly, ordinary oral delivery of glutathione, the most powerful intracellular cancer prevention agent our bodies make, is incredibly hindered by its breakdown in the stomach. In one investigation of 40 healthy adults, supplementation with oral glutathione had no impact on blood levels of the cell reinforcement, and no huge changes were seen in biomarkers of oxidative stress.

To offer medical advantages, nutrients and minerals need to arrive at the objective tissue of activity. Bioavailability is key for supplements and practical nourishments and related wellbeing claims. Many elements influence bioavailability—including stomach related issues, low stomach corrosive, low take-up of a supplement. What's more, supplements themselves fluctuate in the measures of nutrients, minerals and cell reinforcements they offer—some offer more than the suggested day by day sum, some less. Items are sold in various structures (powders, fluids, tablets, containers, chewable, and sticky confections), all of which bring about factor sums. As indicated by one study:" Many ingredients in adult MVMs had mean rate contrasts that were above name guarantees and were profoundly factor between singular items in a representative sampling of the US market."

Enter Liposomal Delivery Systems: Taking a Cue from Nature

The starburst of complex life we see surrounding us consistently started with single cells 3.8 billion years prior—basic, free-floating microorganisms that were one of life's soonest and most keen innovations.

Those basic cells, much the same as our cells today, had a layer made out of a lipid bilayer. The membrane played out a wide range of unprecedented accomplishments: in addition to the fact that it protected within the cell, it permitted supplements to go through and squanders and poisons to be removed. Also, it advanced the ability to convey electricity and to store vitality as ATP atoms. Generally made out of phospholipids, the cell layer was not just defensive, it was exceptionally active

Quick forward to the 1960s, when smart researchers started to try different things with liposomal delivery of medications. Liposomes are minor phospholipid rises with a bilayer structure fundamentally the same as that of our cell membranes. Liposomes end up being perfect transporters for remedial atoms, profoundly viable at conveying supplements straightforwardly into the cell. Liposomes are profoundly biocompatible, and they are fit for holding either water-solvent or fat-dissolvable molecules. Their size, electrical charge, and surfaces can be changed in a lab. Liposomal delivery frameworks have been utilized effectively in clinical preliminaries for an amazing assortment of therapeutics—conveying everything from anticancer to antifungal, calming and antitoxin meds just as complex quality drugs and vaccines.

Liposomal supplements offer a nutritional delivery framework with quick take-up and compelling delivery into the cells. Liposomes are exceptionally effective regarding encouraging cell antioxidant delivery because they are set up from normal phospholipids, they are biocompatible and nontoxic. The liposomal delivery system is getting progressively well known for nutraceuticals because they protect these therapeutic molecules from a breakdown in the stomach related framework. In cell culture considers, liposomes can increment intracellular conveyance 100-fold over non-liposomal delivery.

Liposomal nutraceuticals and wellbeing supplements offer numerous advantages over typical oral formulation. These include:

- High bioavailability and assimilation
- Ensuring supplements against the unforgiving condition of the GI tract
- Expanding oral take-up in the mouth using the mucosa
- Expanded take-up into cells
- Liposomes can be defined to hold both water-solvent and fat
- The fluid organization of liposomes might be progressively perfect for the individuals who experience trouble swallowing huge tablets

Size Matters—And Small is Better

Not all liposomes are indistinguishable. Littler liposomes are far likelier to endure and convey their therapeutic molecules. These littler liposomes offer the fastest take-up and are less handily rummaged and cleared by our immune frameworks. The liposomal delivery system normally falls into three categories:

- MLV (Multi-Lamellar Vesicles) are around 500-5000nm (nanomolar) and have more than one bilayer.
- LUV (Large Unilamellar Vesicles) are ~200-800nm with a solitary bilayer.
- SUV (Small Unilamellar Vesicles) run from 20-150nm and have a long circulation half-life and better cellular delivery over bigger particles.

The ultra-small, unilamellar liposomes are made with modern high-shear equipment. The outcome is firmly controlled, tiny vesicles that are the size of nanoparticles. The littlest, unilamellar (one layer) liposomes flow in the blood the longest and are generally steady. Cell take-up is extraordinarily expanded—as much as multiple times—as liposome size reductions from 236nm down to 97nm. At the littlest size (64 nm), uptake is 34 times higher.

Lipid nanoparticle delivery system has been appeared to significantly improve the ingestion of numerous regular substances, for example, DIM (Diindolylmethane) and milk thistle, which are known to have poor bioavailability on their own. Nanoparticle liposomes are perfect for the delivery of various atoms, particularly when longer-term impacts are attractive.

A Closer Look at Liposomal Supplements

Glutathione benefits drastically from liposomal formulations. Liposomal glutathione can reestablish immune system responses. Liposomal technology is likewise eminently fit a water-dissolvable cancer prevention agent like Vitamin C, expanding blood levels over standard oral supplements. Coenzyme Q10, our most powerful lipid-solvent cell reinforcement, additionally profits by liposomal formulation. Top-notch complex blends of unadulterated mixes and botanicals exacerbated into liposomal plans offer brilliant viability and simplicity of use.

Albeit numerous liposomal products guarantee improved bioavailability, few can convey the expanded retention these formulations can offer. With modern, all around planned, lipid nanoparticle delivery frameworks, the bioavailability, retention and cell take-up of numerous characteristic substances can be significantly improved. Furthermore, as a side advantage, phosphatidylcholine, which makes the layer out of lipid nanoparticles, likewise supports the lipid films of cells, giving phospholipids that can be utilized for cell repair.

The most effective method to Make Liposomal Vitamin C-The Recipe!

I have partitioned the recipe into 5 quick steps that you can utilize.

STEP 1: Take a major container and disintegrate 2 tablespoons ascorbic acid in 1 cup water (great freshwater as in water or spring water).

STEP 2: Take another container, put 6 and a 1/2 Tablespoon lecithin granules in 2 cups of spring water... Save the solution aside for at any rate of two hours.

I incline toward doing steps one and two in the first part of the day with the goal that I give enough time for the lecithin to soak.

STEP 3: Add ascorbic acid water to lecithin water and mix it for a couple of moments to combine.

STEP 4: Pour the blend into Ultra Sonic more cleanly. Turn cleaner on and with spatula move the fluid to and fro ceaselessly in the Ultra Sonic cleaner for 8 minutes. Turn the machine off and tap.

STEP 5: Store the solution in the glass. Not at all like the Water Kefir that we arranged a week ago, the arrangement can't. Keep your drink in the freezer it will be useful for about a month. Drink the solution cold.

Additional TIP: If Liposomal Vitamin C truly tastes severe or it makes a strange sensation on your tongue, at that point it may demonstrate the need for Vitamin C in your body.

I prefer Liposomal Vitamin C to expand my vitality. I realize it is expanding my immune system, do your examination. I take it when I believe I am a piece run down, I am not engrossing my nourishment well, I am in a surge, I am pushed, and so on.- so this prompts me to take Liposomal Vitamin C for at any rate 3-4 times in a day.

Liquid lecithin and liquid vitamin C recipe

I used to make Liposomal Vitamin C in an ultrasonic cleaner and it used to have vodka as a fixing ($$$), and it used to be so tedious that I could never place the time in except if there was a genuine disease to fight. But, during an intense disease is actually when I can't bear to invest the energy. Everywhere throughout the Internet, you can locate that different quality and I feel that they make a quality item. Yet, there's some uplifting news!

In a standard blender, you can make great liposomal nutrient C!

This recipe is from a dear companion and we have both utilized it for ourselves as well as other people to extraordinary impact. The stunt is that lecithin needs to shape liposomes, so the procedure need not be convoluted or difficult. In any case, my encounters with the yield of this recipe have been comparable to those increasingly "advanced" adaptations, so I see no bit of leeway to heading off to all the difficulty.

While my ultrasonic jewelry cleaner accumulates dust, I can make this consistently!

Simple Blender Lipo C

- 6 tablespoons Sunflower Lecithin or Organic Soy Lecithin Powder
- 3 tablespoons Sodium Ascorbate Powder
- 1 cup distilled water

Join all ingredients in a blender container and mix on rapid (or low for a pro-style blender) for at least five minutes, yet no longer than seven minutes. (I have not tried this recipe in a pro-style blender, so your mileage may change.) The recipe might be multiplied, however, I have not tried bunches bigger than that.

Every tablespoon of this liposomal C contains around 1000 mg Vitamin C.

A few people make their lipo C with ascorbic acid powder. I have not tried this variety either, yet I have it on great power that it is a successful recipe and won't antagonistically influence body pH.

Disclaimer: As with anything, continue with caution, ask your doctor.

Chapter 5

The Great Vitamin C HOAX

What do you think Vitamin C is for?

The amount Vitamin C is sufficient and what amount is excessive?

What does Vitamin C do?

A great many people that I pose these questions will say something like this...

"Vitamin C is for your safe framework to treat or forestall colds and flu"

"take however much as could be expected" or "I take until my gut goes interesting" or "1 or 2 grams consistently or each couple of hours when debilitated"

"Nutrient C fixes/forestalls scurvy"

Vitamin C is the greatest hoax on display throughout the entire existence of current medication. Vitamin C is potentially the most widely contemplated vitamin, nutraceutical, corresponding/normal medication ever. We have more logical information on vitamin C than some other fixing. The science is strong and the information is of magnificent quality and the ends in the white paper diary articles are genuine. Right now; lie is spread by the victim of the hoax. It is an insane circumstance where an untruth or a theory can get right the world over before reality gets its jeans on. It is the overall population with old, wrong data, suppositions, and advertising one-liners and "naturopathic" decides and recounted reports that are demanding to utilize nutrient C at an inappropriate portion for an inappropriate explanation. Right now fabrication can't and engendered by "the man" or "big pharma" they are simply providing the interest.

Nobody needs to conceal information or make fake science because the overall population is driving the nutrient C market and development. They need more! Since more is better! Correct? Wrong. What's more, on account of vitamin C the genuine test is keeping the levels at the ideal level; excessively little or a lot of is terrible for you. What's more, moreover Vitamin C needs different supplements and cofactors (nutrients An, E, D, zinc, and bioflavonoids) in the right equalization for it to work at its ideal level.

The Vitamin C story

Scurvy was found. Vitamin c deficiency was seen as the reason for scurvy. The term ascorbic corrosive is gotten from hostile to scorbutic, which means against the scurvy compound. Vitamin C deficiency was connected to low admission because of poor nourishment decisions, poor cultivating practices, and nourishment preparing.

The requirement for vitamin C in the eating routine of people is the consequence of a characteristic mistake in starch digestion. Most animals can combine ascorbic acid from glucose; people, different primates and guinea pigs do not have the catalyst required to make it.

vitamins have consistently been overcome with the belief that they are fundamental and can just do beneficial things with almost no or no toxicities even at supraphysiological portions. The "more is better" philosophy is empowered and reactions are excused.

Curiously with such a great amount of research on vitamin C over such a large number of years demonstrating irrelevant impacts from supplementation at portions past what is important to address lacks the standard dosages utilized by everybody far surpass what the science says we need. Moreover examine shows that vitamin C supplementation more noteworthy than 100-250mg every day for illness avoidance at dosages as meager as 500mg day by day can contribute irrelevantly and at times negative outcomes for a cardiovascular ailment, malignancy, aging, and all-cause mortality.

Indeed, even with these new revelations in the open area high portion enhancements of different types of vitamin C are promptly bought over the counter and with support or solution from medicinal services experts and devoured by the overall population and with the presumption that it is without hazard and liberated from symptoms implies that the negative impacts are generally excused or ascribed to something different.

So what does Vitamin C do?

All known and proposed activities of vitamin C are represented by a solitary synthetic property: ascorbic acid is an electron giver and in this manner a reducing agent. The most very much described activities are those as a chemical cofactor, incorporating those in which it is a genuine co-substrate.

Physiological elements of vitamin C (L-ascorbic corrosive) include:

- Investment in hydroxylation responses: collagen creation, tyrosine, noradrenaline and serotonin, just as L-Carnitine, steroid hormones of the adrenal organs and bile acids.

- The collagen production function is to encourage the hydroxylation of proline and lysine buildups in collagen, permitting legitimate intracellular collapsing of professional collagen for fare and testimony as developing collagen. Normal side effects of scurvy incorporate injury dehiscence, poor injury recuperating and relaxing of teeth, all highlighting abandons in connective tissue. Collagen gives connective tissue structural strength.

- Ascorbic acid and stress – it has been notable since the 1920's that the adrenal gland has elevated levels and exceptionally dynamic take-up of vitamin C. Beforehand it was accepted that vitamin c was essential for cortisol creation yet that has been disproven. Proposals that vitamin C can be an enemy of stress compound and right adrenal weariness or adrenal weakness are additionally deceptive. In the adrenal gland, vitamin C works in both the chromaffin cell arrangement of the adrenal medulla and adrenal cortex. Dopamine b-hydroxylase, found in neurosecretory vesicles and adrenal chromaffin granules in the adrenal medulla is vital for the union of norepinephrine from dopamine in the nervous system and the adrenal organs. Nutrient C additionally animates catecholamine discharge using the NO-initiated component. During stress nutrient c assists with balancing the hepatic and adrenal CYP450 specifically CYP45011B that directs aldosterone creation and release for controlling sodium levels. The cancer prevention agent impacts of vitamin C are defensive to cell structures during expanded physical and mental interest.

- Ascorbate has likewise been appeared to aid the hydroxylation of hypoxia-inducible factor 1α (HIF-1α). HIF-1α is a transcription factor liable for the cell reaction to low oxygen conditions through the initiation of qualities controlling differing cell pathways including glycolysis, iron vehicle, angiogenesis, and cell endurance.

- As a reducer, it takes an interest in biosynthesis of tetrahydrofolic acid (an initiated type of folic acid), hyaluronic corrosive (for collagen, joint, and ligament) and prostaglandins (aggravation and circulation)

- It likewise adjusts the body's invulnerability by invigorating the creation of immunoglobulins and interferons

- Cell reinforcement Vitamin C is effectively and reversibly oxidized into dehydro-L-ascorbic corrosive, making a redox framework that permits it to go about as a cancer prevention agent. It deactivates numerous ROS. It additionally recovers nutrient E spent during comparable procedures. In this way, nutrient C assumes a significant job in disposing of oxidative pressure which, in the mix with its water solvency, makes it the cancer prevention agent of extracellular liquids.

- Ace oxidant ascorbate can decrease metals, for example, copper and iron, prompting the development of superoxide and hydrogen peroxide, and resulting in an age of receptive oxidant species.
- Vitamin C additionally partakes in detoxification of xenobiotics adding to the production of ROS
- Peptidylglycine an amidating monooxygenase, found in secretory vesicles is required to amidated numerous peptide hormones to make them organically dynamic. These incorporate numerous hypothalamic and gastrointestinal hormones, for example, gastrin, cholecystokinin, calcitonin, vasopressin, and oxytocin;
- L-Carnitine synthesis – Trimethyllysine hydroxylase and c-butyrobetaine hydroxylases are required for carnitine blend from the fundamental amino acids lysine and methionine. The enzymes require iron, alpha-ketoglutarate, and a reductant, of which ascorbate is the most ideal.
- 4-Hydroxyphenylpyruvate dioxygenase is required for the catabolism of tyrosine. Ascorbate lack prompts debilitated tyrosine catabolism and expanded plasma groupings of tyrosine.

- Components of the cancer prevention agent framework, which are required for the integrity of immune cells since they are dependent upon a high weight of reactive oxygen species (ROS)
- The hydroxylation of tryptophan in serotonin biosynthesis;
- The union of catecholamines;
- Detoxification of various substances in the liver by animating the blend of cytochrome P450,
- A job in iron exchange from the iron moving protein transferrin to the iron stockpiling protein ferritin, the advancement of intestinal iron retention by lessening almost non-absorbable Fe^{3+} to all the more effectively absorbable Fe^{2+} and by repressing the creation of insoluble iron-tannin and iron-phytate complexes,
- Ascorbate is proposed as a neuromodulator of glutamatergic, dopaminergic, cholinergic and GABAergic transmission and related practices.

Cancer prevention agent or pro-oxidant?

Artificially, nutrient C is an electron donor or lessening operator, and electrons from ascorbate represent the entirety of its known physiological impacts.

Vitamin C is called a cell reinforcement since electrons from vitamin C can lessen oxidized species or oxidants. Notwithstanding, similar electrons from ascorbate can decrease metals, for example, copper and iron, prompting arrangement of superoxide and hydrogen peroxide, and consequent age of receptive oxidant species. Along these lines, under certain conditions ascorbate, is a pro-oxidant.

What amount would it be a good idea for me to utilize?

The impact of a single oral dose of vitamin C on the intracellular ascorbate grouping of immunocompetent cells, similar to monocytes and neutrophils, is described by a sigmoidal reaction bend. In adults, a vitamin C intake of roughly 100 mg/d brings about complete intracellular saturation.

What amount is excessive?

Vitamin C is non-toxic, be that as it may, its enormous dosages (500 mg/d or more) can cause nutritious tract unsettling influences (queasiness, pyrosis, and diarrhea), improved urine with a sentiment of consuming, and erythrocyte hemolysis during glucose-6-phosphate dehydrogenase (G-6-PD) and vitamin B12 inadequacy. To place this in context the vast majority focus on 1000mg per portion with 2000 to 6000mg every day being a typical portion. 500mg every day is a generally low portion for vitamin C supplements.

By initiating extreme pee fermentation, such portions hinder the excretion of weak acids and bases, which may bring about the precipitation of cystine and urate depositions in the urinary tract, prompting the arrangement of renal calculi. Vitamin C portions > 1g/d lift blood and urinary oxalic corrosive focuses on a degree expanding the risk of calculi development from calcium oxalate. In this manner, such enormous portions ought not to be controlled in interminable renal failure, cystinuria, the inclination to gout, urate and oxalate calculosis. Restoratively applied vitamin C expands blood sodium fixation and diminishes potassium focus which can prompt inadequacy of the last mentioned. Likewise, it contrarily impacts on certain medications taken, causing vitamin B12 annihilation (along these lines, the two vitamins ought not to be directed in the mix), and enlarges amphetamine subsidiary and tricyclic energizer sedate end by repressing their reabsorption in renal tubules. Because of its chemical compatibility, vitamin C ought not to be regulated with drugs that have oxidizing properties. By acidifying the urine, it can prompt the crystallization of urine released p-aminosalicylic corrosive and sulphonamides. The utilization of high-portion vitamin C yields bogus outcomes in body liquid investigations performed with the utilization of techniques dependent on redox responses, for example, determinations of bilirubin, glucose, or creatinine focuses, and LDH or AspAT activity.

High portions of vitamin C hamper copper ingestion and inhibit copper-containing ceruloplasmin and superoxide dismutase (Cu, Zn-SOD) activities. Interestingly, they upgrade iron assimilation to an unsafe degree in people with its exorbitant intestinal retention, and in those with expanded blood iron focus, and with hemochromatosis, sideroblastic anemia or thalassemia (where the side effects intensify. The excess unbound iron collects in the tissues and skin, disturbs gastrointestinal mucosa, causes inebriation, and adds to the prooxidant impacts of vitamin C.

Chapter 6

Myths and Facts about Vitamin C

A great many people know some things about vitamin C, similar to that it's in oranges, or that without it you can create scurvy (as sailors broadly did). Yet, myths about this fundamental nutrient are additionally still genuinely normal, and the fact of the matter is our insight about its advantages and capacities keeps on developing.

For instance, did you realize that vitamin C may support your cardiovascular wellbeing? An investigation from the University of Colorado, Boulder, found that that a 500-milligram time-released portion of vitamin C protectively affected veins that were like a walking workout, provoking some to dub vitamin C the "exercise pill."

Presently, I wouldn't go that far: The investigation was little, including only 35 inactive overweight or obese adults, and the reasons to practice go past vein wellbeing. Yet, this unquestionably proposes vitamin C does unmistakably more for our bodies than support immunity.

What else don't you think about vitamin C? Test your nourishment IQ with my five fantasies and realities about this entrancing nutrient.

Myth: Blasting a cold with vitamin C will fight it off

Since cold and flu season is authoritatively increasing, many individuals are stacking up on OJ and vitamin C enhancements to abstain from becoming ill. Yet, tragically, that may not be as gainful as you might suspect.

While some examination shows that individuals who routinely take vitamin C enhancements may have marginally shorter colds or fairly milder manifestations, for a great many people, boosting vitamin C doesn't lessen the danger of coming down with the regular bug. I state "a great many people" because there are examines that show that vitamin C cut cold risk in 50% male athletes, yet not in females.

The facts confirm that vitamin C is basic for safe capacity and that it assumes a key job in wound mending. However, the most ideal approach to keep your immune system strong is to eat restoratively, including vitamin C-rich produce, constantly. Lamentably, the most recent details show that 90% of Americans fall short of the prescribed least 1½ to 2 day by day cups of foods grown from the ground to 3 everyday cups of veggies. Fill that gap and you'll effectively take in any event 200 milligrams of nutrient C day by day, enough to keep your invulnerable framework very much upheld consistently so you won't have to play make up for a lost time.

Fact: Vitamin C deficiencies are rare

Our bodies can't create nutrient C, which is the thing that makes this supplement fundamental, which means we should acquire it from nourishment. However, nowadays a lack sufficiently genuine to cause side effects, which can incorporate draining gums and nosebleeds, swollen joints, unpleasant, dry skin, and wounding, is uncommon.

The suggested day by day focus for grown-ups is 75 milligrams for ladies, and 90 for men, albeit numerous specialists trust it ought to be raised to 200 milligrams, the sum that immerses the body's tissues. One medium orange gives around 70 milligrams, and scurvy can be forestalled with as meager as 10 every day milligrams of vitamin C. As it were, you're most likely not at risk of a genuine insufficiency; however, that doesn't mean you shouldn't endeavor to get enough.

Myth: Citrus is the best source of vitamin C

While citrus is a fantastic wellspring of vitamin C, a veggie—chime peppers—proves to be the best. One cup of chopped raw red chime pepper (about the size of a tennis ball) packs 200 to 300 milligrams of vitamin C, around 100 over a cup of OJ. Other great sources incorporate broccoli, Brussels grows, kiwi, strawberries, papaya, pineapple, and melon, just as (obviously) citrus natural products, similar to oranges, tangerines, and grapefruit.

Fact: Adequate vitamin C intake helps weight loss: certainty

A low blood level of vitamin C has been connected to having a higher BMI, muscle versus fat ratio, and waist circumference, contrasted with individuals with ordinary levels. Furthermore, an investigation from Arizona State University found that vitamin C status may influence the body's capacity to utilize fat as a fuel source during both exercise and rest.

To receive nutrient C's weight control rewards your most logical option is to concentrate on being dynamic and making your suppers with beautiful produce that is normally plentiful in vitamin C.

Myth: You can't get an excessive amount of vitamin C

Your body can't store vitamin C, so when you expend more than you need, the surplus is disposed of by your kidneys in urine. That doesn't mean, in any case, that enormous portions can't make unwanted symptoms. Nutrient C is one of the supplements that have a set up Tolerable Upper Intake Level or UL the most extreme prompted consumption, from both nourishment and enhancements joined.

For vitamin C it's 2,000 milligrams every day, and keeping in mind that a few people might be fine taking right now more, megadoses of vitamin C supplements have been appeared to trigger swelling and stomach related bombshell, diarrhea, queasiness, regurgitating, heartburn, headache, a sleeping disorder, and kidney stones. Main concern: More unquestionably isn't better; simply enough is in certainty spot on!

Which nutrients do liposomes have the most benefits?

At the point when a functioning substance is embodied in a liposome, it very well may be shielded from quick debasement and disposal in the body. The substance is consequently ready to circle inside the body for a more extended timeframe. This will improve the probability that the active substance will enter the objective tissues and cells. Research has additionally demonstrated that beyond what one substance can be stacked into a liposome to make them work synergistically.

ENHANCED DELIVERY

There is a wide range of approaches to oversee a liposomal type of a functioning substance, for example by intravenous infusion, nearby infusion, inward breath yet also by simple oral intake. While the organization of liposomal meds into the circulation system can be an unmistakable and direct approach to target unhealthy destinations in the body, the oral organization is frequently best as a less intrusive organization course. The detriment of the oral course is that the liposomes need to go through the stomach and digestive system, which structure a generally antagonistic condition influencing the solidness of liposomal items. A lot of research exertion has been embraced to build liposomes that go through the stomach and digestive system in an unblemished structure, demonstrating that at times the organic accessibility of orally controlled active substances can be sure to be improved.

BETTER EFFICACY – LESS TOXICITY

Liposomes are typically made of normally inferred beginning materials. They are basically non-lethal and naturally degradable. They have the exceptional capacity to hold dynamic substances – including meds and enhancements – both in their watery inside just as their lipid bilayer. This makes liposomes appealing as medication delivery frameworks. Medication delivery specifically at unhealthy destinations in the body expands the neighborhood grouping of the medication improving its pharmacologic impact. It has additionally been shown that the liposomal exemplification of a medication can fundamentally decrease its risk by the propensity of liposomes to avoid from solid organs and shield these from exposure to the encapsulated drug.

Protection

Studies uncover that liposomes – tackling their capacity to embody and transport dynamic fixings – can expand the bioavailability and target delivery of these fixings in the body. This impact has been ascribed to:

- liposomal protection of the active substance against enzymatic or hydrolytic corruption as it goes through the stomach and digestive system;
- improved enterocyte association in the digestive system, expanding the convergence of the active substance at the site where it must be taken up;
- prolongation of the 'residence time' of a liposomal exemplified active substance in the body and at the objective site;
- Liposomal redirection of the actives after take-up, shielding the active substance from quick clearance. Numerous active substances that are managed conventionally are essentially lost because after ingestion they are driven directly to the liver (the 'hepatic entry framework'). The liver separates the active substance before it gets the opportunity to arrive at the objective cells.

The liposomal embodiment can help forestall this misfortune.

Vitamin C

Another examination has demonstrated that the intravenous administration of liposomal vitamin C prompts the most noteworthy ascent in vitamin C levels in the blood. The oral organization of liposomal vitamin C prompts marginally lower blood levels of vitamin C, yet even these are still a lot higher than after the oral organization of non-liposomal vitamin C.

IMPROVED UPTAKE

In any case, regardless of whether unblemished entry through the stomach and digestive system can't, liposome items, for example, liposome nutrient enhancements can be of incredible advantage. Particularly lipophilic active substances that have low dissolvability in water, show poor assimilation and in this way second rate adequacy. It has been demonstrated that lipid definitions can fundamentally improve the intestinal take-up of such hard to-plan lipophilic actives.

Why should you not take vitamin supplements?

Over-the-counter dietary enhancements are an enormous business — over 90,000 items create about $30 billion consistently in the United States.

More established grown-ups make up a major piece of these deals, as well. An overview of just about 3,500 grown-ups ages 60, 70% utilize a day by day supplement (either a multivitamin or individual nutrient or mineral), 54% take a couple of enhancements, and 29% take at least four.

However, are these pills acceptable medication, or misuse of cash?

"Supplements are never a substitute for a fair, invigorating eating routine," says Dr. JoAnn Manson, a teacher of medication at Harvard Medical School and educator of the study of disease transmission at Harvard's T.H. Chan School of Public Health. "Furthermore, they can be an interruption from a sound way of life practice that presents a lot more noteworthy advantages."

What science appears

Dietary enhancement is an umbrella term that incorporates everything from nutrients and minerals to botanicals and biosimilar items, (for example, alleged "natural male hormone"). Generally, however, individuals use "supplement" to mean an individual nutrient or mineral arrangement or a multivitamin (that is, an item that contains at least 10 nutrients, minerals, or both).

Even though enhancements are well known, there is restricted proof that they offer any noteworthy medical advantages. Indeed, an investigation distributed online May 28, 2018, by the Journal of the American College of Cardiology, found that the four most normally utilized enhancements — multivitamins, vitamin D, calcium, and vitamin C — didn't ensure against cardiovascular malady.

So for what reason do such a large number of individuals take supplements if the medical advantages are immaterial or nonexistent for the normal, solid individual? "Individuals regularly consider them a bonus they can do to be certain their essential wholesome needs are secured,". There's additionally a potential misleading impact on taking enhancements, she includes. "Individuals feel more advantageous on the off chance that they accomplish something they accept makes them sound."

The best issue with supplements is that they are not controlled by the FDA. "Enhancements can show up on the rack without demonstrating they offer any advantages," says Dr. Manson. "With restricted guideline and oversight, it's additionally hard to know for sure that the enhancement contains the fixings on the mark and is liberated from contaminants."

It's not all awful news, however. For example, some exploration has indicated that folic corrosive and B-complex nutrients may lessen the danger of stroke. Likewise, the Physicians' Health Study II, distributed in 2012 by Harvard scientists, found that men who took a day by day multivitamin for a long time had an 8% lower danger of malignant growth and a 9% lower risk of cataracts contrasted with a placebo group.

Conceivable wellbeing risks

Most enhancements are protected to take, however, there are exemptions. For instance:

- High dosages of beta carotene have been connected to more danger of lung malignant growth in smokers.
- Additional calcium and vitamin D may expand the danger of kidney stones.
- High dosages of vitamin E may prompt stroke brought about by seeping in the cerebrum.
- Vitamin K can meddle with the counter coagulating impacts of blood thinners.
- Taking high measures of vitamin B6 for a year or longer has been related to nerve harm that can weaken body developments (the side effects regularly leave after the enhancements are halted).

A job for high-risk groups

Enhancements can assume a significant job for some high-risk groups. For example, Adults determined to have osteoporosis may require additional nutrient D and calcium past what they get from their regular eating regimen.

Enhancements additionally can help individuals with Crohn's infection or celiac sickness, conditions that make it hard to assimilate certain supplements. Individuals with nutrient B12 lack quite often need an enhancement.

Some examination likewise has discovered that a formula of vitamin C, vitamin E, carotenoids, zinc, and copper can lessen the movement old enough related macular degeneration, a significant reason for vision misfortune among older adults. "Also, individuals who are lactose narrow-minded and don't get enough nutrient D and calcium since they don't eat dairy items additionally could profit by supplements," says Dr. Manson.

The message here is that enhancements endorsed by a specialist are useful for individuals with certain clinical issues. Something else, it's ideal to get your nutrients and minerals from nourishment and not a pill.

Should You Take Dietary Supplements?

At the point when you go after that bottle of vitamin C or fish oil pills, you may think about how well they'll function if they're sheltered. The main thing to ask yourself is whether you need them in any case.

The greater part of all Americans take at least one dietary enhancements every day or once in a while.

Enhancements are accessible without a remedy and typically come in pill, powder or fluid structure. Normal enhancements incorporate nutrients, minerals and herbal products, otherwise called botanicals.

Individuals take these enhancements to ensure they get enough basic supplements and to keep up or improve their wellbeing. But, not every person needs to take supplements.

"It's conceivable to get the entirety of the supplements you need by eating an assortment of solid nourishments, so you don't need to take one," an enlisted dietitian and advisor to NIH. "But, supplements can help fill in holes in your eating routine."

A few Supplements may have reactions, particularly whenever taken before a medical procedure or with different prescriptions. Supplements can likewise cause issues on the off chance that you have certain wellbeing conditions. What's more, the impacts of numerous enhancements haven't been tried in kids, pregnant ladies, and different gatherings. So talk with your social insurance supplier in case you're pondering taking dietary supplements.

"You ought to talk about with your doctor what supplements you're taking so your consideration can be incorporated and overseen,"

Dietary supplements are controlled by the U.S. Food and Drug Administration (FDA) as food sources, not as medications. The name may guarantee certain medical advantages. But, in contrast to meds, supplements can't profess to fix, treat or forestall an infection.

"There's little proof that any supplement can turn around the course of any incessant infection," says Hopp. "Try not to take supplements with that desire."

Proof suggests that a few supplements can upgrade wellbeing in various manners. The most famous supplement supplements are multivitamins, calcium, and vitamins B, C and D. Calcium supports bone wellbeing, and nutrient D enables the body to ingest calcium. Nutrients C and E are cancer prevention agents—atoms that forestall cell harm and help to look after wellbeing.

Ladies need iron during pregnancy, and breastfed babies need nutrient D. Folic corrosive—400 micrograms day by day, regardless of whether from supplements or braced nourishment—is significant for all ladies of childbearing age.

Vitamin B12 keeps nerves and platelets solid. "Nutrient B12, for the most part, originates from meat, fish and dairy nourishments, so veggie lovers may believe taking a supplement to make certain to get enough of it," Haggans says.

The research proposes that fish oil can advance heart wellbeing. Of the enhancements not got from nutrients and minerals, Hopp says, "fish oil likely has the most logical proof to help its utilization."

The wellbeing impacts of some other regular supplements need more examination. These incorporate glucosamine (for joint torment) and homegrown enhancements, for example, echinacea (invulnerable wellbeing) and flaxseed oil (absorption).

Numerous enhancements have mellow impacts with scarcely any dangers. However, use alert. Nutrient K, for instance, will decrease the capacity of blood thinners to work. Ginkgo can build blood diminishing. The herb St. John's wort is now and then used to ease despondency, tension or pain yet it can likewise speed the breakdown of numerous medications, for example, antidepressants and anti-conception medication pills—and make them less compelling.

Because a supplement is advanced as "characteristic" doesn't mean it's sheltered. The herbs comfrey and kava, for instance, can genuinely harm the liver.

"It's imperative to know the concoction cosmetics, how it's readied, and how it works in the body—

particularly for herbs, yet also for supplements," says Haggans. "Converse with a human services supplier for guidance on whether you need enhancement in any case, the portion and potential connections with medication that is no joke."

For vitamins and minerals, check the % Daily Value (DV) for every supplement to ensure you're not getting excessively. "It's critical to think about the DV. A lot of specific supplements can be destructive.

Researchers despite everything have a lot to learn even about regular nutrients. One ongoing examination discovered unforeseen proof about vitamin E. Prior research recommended that men who took vitamin E supplements may have a lower risk of creating prostate malignant growth. "In any case, causing us a deep sense of shock, an enormous NIH-supported clinical preliminary of more than 29,000 men found that taking supplements of vitamin E raised—not diminished—their danger of this malady," says Dr. Paul M. Coates, executive of NIH's Office of Dietary Supplements. That is the reason it's critical to direct clinical investigations of supplements to affirm their belongings.

Since supplements are directed as nourishments, not as medications, the FDA doesn't assess the nature of enhancements or survey their consequences for the body. If a product is seen as perilous after it arrives at the market, the FDA can limit or boycott its utilization.

Makers are additionally answerable for the item's immaculateness, and they should precisely list fixings and their sums. In any case, there's no administrative organization that ensures that names coordinate what's in the jugs. You chance to get less, or some of the time more, of the recorded fixings. The entirety of the fixings may not be recorded.

A couple of free associations lead quality trials of enhancements and offer seals of endorsement. This doesn't ensure the item works or is protected; it just guarantees the item was appropriately made and contains the recorded fixings.

"products sold broadly in the stores and online where you for the most part shop ought to be fine," Coates says. "As indicated by the FDA, supplements products well on the way to be debased with pharmaceutical ingredients are natural cures advanced for weight reduction and sexual or athletic execution upgrade."

Chapter 7

Advantages of liposomal vitamin C

Did you realize that individuals are among just a group of animal types that can't deliver their inventory of Vitamin C?

Vitamin C, being a water-solvent nutrient, is continually moved out of the body if it isn't being utilized, so ordinary admission of nourishments plentiful in Vitamin C is basic to wellbeing, as found by mariners a couple of hundred years back. The stresses of the present day can imply that more Vitamin C is being required, so expanding our utilization is significant, when this ground-breaking supplement is utilized by such a large number of various pieces of the body and has numerous significant jobs.

There are numerous kinds of Vitamin C supplements accessible, however, Liposomal Vitamin C is the first choice of individuals who truly comprehend bio-accessibility and the significance of high-portion vitamin C. So what sets Liposomal Vitamin C separated from different types of vitamin C that we might be taking to help support our wellbeing? Right off the bat, every single other type of vitamin C face a retention hindrance that inconceivably confines the degree of nutrient C that can enter the circulation system. The enormous measure of nutrient C that doesn't get consumed, gets flushed. In any case, Liposomal Vitamin C adequately slips over the intestinal divider and into the blood.

This sort of Vitamin C likewise doesn't get separated until it arrives at the piece of the body that needs it most. That is because it can sidestep the limitations of the vehicle framework that drastically restrains the bio-accessibility of all non-liposome types of vitamin C. Late clinical preliminaries propose that Liposomal Vitamin C can deliver serum levels of nutrient C about twofold those idea hypothetically conceivable with any oral type of vitamin C.

Traditional types of Vitamin C seriously limit the sum you can take orally. If you take multiple or 2 grams of traditional Vitamin C, the ascorbic acid in the digestive organs will cause gastric trouble including gas, spasms, and the runs. A significant part of Vitamin C will be dispensed within the free stool and the pee. A rate (as meager as 12%) of normal Vitamin C gets retained into the circulation system. The human digestive system was never intended to process enormous dosages of Vitamin C in any structure orally!

However, Liposomal Vitamin C permits you to take Vitamin C orally, sidestep the stomach related framework and convey it crisp and unblemished into the circulatory system. Using "Liposomal Encapsulation Technology"(LET), it fundamentally changes how Vitamin C is conveyed to the circulation system.

There is no framework, organ, organ or cell in your body which doesn't possibly get extraordinary benefit from an optimal supply of Vitamin C. If dietary Vitamin C intake is insufficient, all might be significantly fortified by supplementation with a non-degraded Vitamin C, for example, Liposomal Vitamin C.

Advantages

Powerful Anti-Aging†
Recent considers are demonstrating vitamin C's amazing enemy of maturing benefits. Vitamin C can't a significant enemy of oxidant, a more straightforward advantage is that it controls and advances collagen creation in the body. Hair, nail, skin, bone, heart, teeth and joint wellbeing, indeed, wellbeing for all zones of the body straightforwardly identify with your capacity to deliver collagen. Studies show that vitamin C (ascorbic acid) can expand collagen creation by 8-fold! Lipo Naturals Sunflower Liposomal C raises levels of vitamin C in your organs and regions of the body not already conceivable without direct intravenous (IV vitamin C) infusion.

At the point when first beginning Lipo Naturals Sunflower Liposomal C, you'll notice an improvement in your nail wellbeing, skin composition, and versatility. Some observe sensational enhancements in just a month. Regular utilization will uncover increasingly against maturing benefits, the hair will be more grounded and shinier while forestalling maturing's impacts on the body. As we age, significant levels of vitamin C likewise ensure brain and cardiovascular wellbeing, forestalling age-related degeneration.

Boost Immunity†

Most warm-blooded animals produce vitamin C, aside from humans. Did you realize that most vertebrates produce their vitamin C? In light of what is accepted to be a hereditary transformation in our precursors, people are one of the not many well-evolved creatures who must get nutrient C from their eating regimen. A typical 155lb well-evolved creature will deliver about 13,000mg of vitamin C in their blood every day. Significantly (more than 10x this sum) is delivered whenever harmed, focused or fighting disease.

Late examinations demonstrate a strong link to vitamin C levels and regular immune function. Most researchers will concede, we don't have the idea about all the advantages starting at yet. High dosages of vitamin C (sometimes called megadoses) are indicating amazing outcomes for helping support the body's immune system. Vitamin C raises hydrogen peroxide levels that pathogens and unfortunate cells are helpless against, leaving solid human cells, who endure the higher peroxide levels, safe. Vitamin C seems to be the body's regular resistance against awful entertainers, and we are just barely finding the advantages.

Improve Energy Levels†

Vitamin C is known to help vitality levels in both significant level competitors and people with regular activity levels. An ongoing report shows that elevated levels of vitamin C decreased business-related weakness in any case typically solid subjects. This implies, regardless of whether your vitality levels are acceptable now, you will at a present profit by a high portion of vitamin C. if you have an evening 'disquietude,' and inconvenience focusing as the day goes on, our Sunflower Liposomal C will help.

If you work out, not long after beginning Lipo Naturals Sunflower Liposomal C, you'll notice that you'll have the option to practice longer with less strain... expanding your stamina drastically. Our clients have said they inhale less intensely while practicing longer.

Conclusion

Thank you for making it through to the end of *How to Make Liposomal Vitamin C at Home.* We hope it was informative and able to provide you with all the tools you need to achieve your goals - whatever they are.

Did you enjoy this book?

If you found this book useful, a review on Amazon would be much appreciated.